Christian Journal for Women with Anxiety

christian journal
for women with anxiety

Prompts to Soothe
Anxious Thoughts and Find
Strength in Your Faith

SHAWN HORN, PsyD

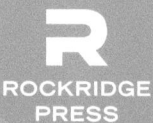

ROCKRIDGE
PRESS

No book, including this one, can ever replace the diagnostic expertise and medical advice of a physician in providing information about your health. The information contained herein is not intended to replace medical advice. You should consult with your doctor before using the information in this or any health-related book.

As of press time, the URLs in this book link or refer to existing websites on the internet. Rockridge Press is not responsible for the outdated, inaccurate, or incomplete content available on these sites.

Unless otherwise indicated, all Scripture quotations are taken from the Holy Bible, New International Version®, NIV®. Copyright © 1973, 1978, 1984, 2011 by Biblica Inc.® Used by permission. All rights reserved worldwide. All other quoted material is in the public domain.

Copyright © 2022 by Rockridge Press

All rights reserved. No part of this publication may be reproduced, stored in a retrieval system, or transmitted in any form or by any means, electronic, mechanical, photocopying, recording, scanning, or otherwise without the prior written permission of the Publisher. Requests to the Publisher for permission should be addressed to the Permissions Department, Rockridge Press, 1955 Broadway, Suite 400, Oakland, CA 94612.

First Rockridge Press trade paperback edition 2022

Rockridge Press and the Rockridge Press logo are trademarks or registered trademarks of Callisto Media Inc. and/or its affiliates in the United States and other countries and may not be used without written permission.

For general information on our other products and services, please contact our Customer Care Department within the United States at (866) 744-2665, or outside the United States at (510) 253-0500.

Paperback ISBN: 978-1-63878-568-2

Manufactured in the United States of America

Interior and Cover Designer: Stephanie Mautone
Art Producer: Megan Baggott
Editor: Carolyn Abate
Production Editor: Emily Sheehan
Production Manager: Riley Hoffman

Author photo courtesy of Nichole Mischke Media

10 9 8 7 6 5 4 3 2 1 0

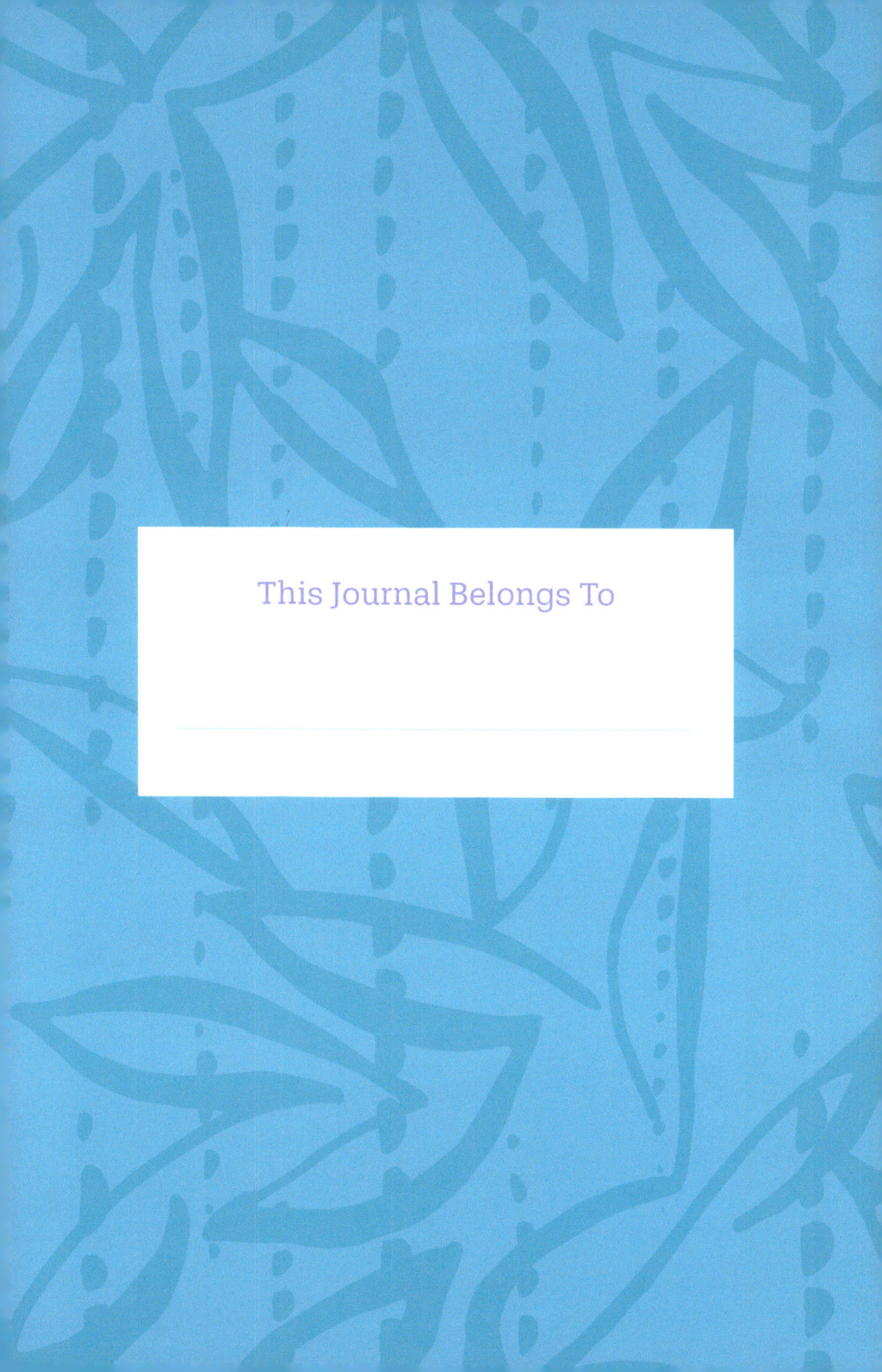

Contents

Introduction **viii** | How to Use This Journal **xi**
A Brief Word on Anxiety **xii**

I   Seek Peace for Your Anxiety
through Your Faith   **1**

II   Challenge Negative Thinking
with Biblical Wisdom   **25**

III   Nurture Your Emotional and
Physical Well-Being   **49**

IV   Look Beyond Prayer for Relief   **69**

V   Self-Care through God's Love   **87**

IV   Calm Anxiety with a Grateful Heart   **107**

Continue Your Healing Journey with Faith **127**
Resources **132** | References **134**

Introduction

Imagine a peaceful, supportive, and safe healing space where you can go every day to quiet your mind, renew your spirit, and be with God.

Wouldn't that be amazing?

The idea of a calm, quiet mind may seem out of reach. The anxious mind is rarely still and present. It's usually busy ruminating on the past, worrying about the future, and anticipating impending doom. I call this overfunctioning for other people's dysfunction, or trying to control that which it cannot control. Exhausting, right?

As a Christian, you've likely been told, "Don't be anxious . . . rest in God." But in many areas of your life, including your physical and mental health, you need more than a mindset or prayer alone—you also benefit from helpful resources and interventions. That doesn't mean you are turning away from God. On the contrary, your intimate relationship with God is the ultimate holding space for you to assess and work through your burdens and struggles.

It is my mission, as a Christian and a psychologist, to help individuals remove the psychological obstacles that are inhibiting their spiritual growth. Research shows that integrating mental health treatment with a person's religious beliefs has better outcomes than treatment alone. It also can strengthen your faith and facilitate spiritual growth. I wrote this faith-based integrated guided journal with you in mind. Think of it as a resource that integrates Bible-based fundamentals with evidence-based tools so you can better manage anxiety, deepen your faith, and strengthen your relationship with God.

I come to this book with over two decades of experience in the management and treatment of anxiety disorders. And, from the wisdom and understanding that comes from the Christian journey and biblical training. I earned a bachelor's degree in psychology at Seattle Pacific University and hold a doctorate in clinical psychology from George Fox University, where I also received seminary training in biblical studies and spiritual formation.

This journal is for Christian women of all backgrounds, experiences, and denominations. In this journal you'll find a host of prompts, practices, and exercises to help you reflect, focus, and take action to mitigate your anxiety. It is all presented in a way that keeps your faith front and center so you can find comfort and hope as you embark on this journey.

My hope is that this journal will be a useful tool in supporting that mission and offer you a peaceful, safe space to pause, reflect, heal, and grow.

So, let's get started!

How to Use This Journal

This journal is organized into six sections, each containing relevant journal prompts, Bible verses, and life application practices. The journal prompts facilitate a deeper dive into your healing journey by encouraging you to reflect and write on posed questions or statements. The Bible verses offer spiritual application for masterful living. Finally, the life application practices offer specific strategies and tools for emotional well-being, personal development, and spiritual growth.

These three components, applied together, offer an integrated approach to anxiety management. You can start from the beginning or flip to specific topics and practices depending on your needs and time considerations. Although this journal is a helpful tool, it's not a replacement for treatment. Any ongoing or debilitating feelings of depression or anxiety should be addressed by a medical professional. They can evaluate your individual situation and create a personalized treatment plan appropriate for your specific needs.

Before beginning, I want to congratulate you for setting the intention to improve your emotional, personal, and spiritual health, and always remember:

Healing is possible, and hope is a promise.

A Brief Word on Anxiety

Anxiety is a normal part of your emotional experience. It motivates you, alerts you of potential danger, and fuels your body with specific chemical messengers required for fast reaction in emergencies. It reminds you to take care of your responsibilities when you are avoiding them or nags at you when you are doing something you shouldn't. In many of these instances, anxiety is adaptive and necessary. It becomes maladaptive when it begins to negatively impact a person's life and daily functioning. Today, anxiety is the most common mental health disorder in the United States. Even though it is so prevalent, many remain silent and suffer alone.

Historically, we tend to shame, blame, and stigmatize that which we don't understand. Because of the lack of understanding, many people have been tragically accused of causing their own struggles; doing something wrong; not having enough faith, prayer, or belief; or refusing to change. It's time to clear this up. There is no shame in having anxiety. You're not alone. It's not your fault, and it isn't even what you think. God is neither punishing you nor abandoning you.

When it comes to understanding and treating anxiety, there is a need to address the tissues (biophysiology) to work on the issues (psychology). This means anxiety is part of your ancient survival brain response and will unconsciously and involuntarily activate when danger is detected. That's worth repeating. Anxiety will *unconsciously* and *involuntarily activate* under the right conditions with the right variables. Let that soak in for a moment. You aren't choosing this! When anxiety is activated, the fight or flight nervous system response will override your higher cognitive functions (logic, reason, reframing, challenging irrational thoughts, having the bigger perspective, and more). That explains why it may feel nearly impossible to *think* your way out of anxiety.

Recent findings in neuroscience provide a deeper understanding of why there is a tendency to become stuck in the anxious response and offers new tips and tricks to get unstuck, especially when it is a challenge to do so with thought alone. The practices and information in this guided journal are based on the science that offers hope for new possibilities, with new perspectives for your healing journey.

I

Seek Peace for Your Anxiety through Your Faith

Anxiety is an internal alarm, hardwired into your nervous system, alerting you of potential danger and signaling for an appropriate behavioral response. The longer you ignore or resist your internal alarm, the worse it gets over time, becoming louder, like it's saying, "Do you hear me now?!" If you don't understand what anxiety is trying to communicate, and/or lack the proper skills to attend to the alarm, you are at risk of maladaptive responses and coping skills.

Let's begin the healing journey by tapping into the soothing power of faith. Faith is your assurance and hope that God is present, has the power to help, and is attending to the alarm. This section will provide you with an opportunity to explore how faith can offer a new sense of peace during your anxiety alarm. It also will explore specific evidence-based tools to put faith into action.

But those who hope in the Lord *will renew their strength. They will soar on wings like eagles; They will run and not grow weary; they will walk and not be faint.*

ISAIAH 40:31 (NIV)

Notice Isaiah 40:31 does not say God will *remove* the struggle; it states He will *renew* your strength. Faith, if based on the expectation and requirement for emotional relief, will not sustain. Faith gives you strength to tolerate distress by turning your focus from pain toward a focus on God. Meditating on His promises, presence, love, etc. will give you strength. Write about a time in your life when your faith and hope renewed your strength and helped you overcome a seemingly impossible barrier.

Some describe faith not as something you have but as a relationship you are in. Having faith in God involves an attunement to His presence in your everyday experiences. How have you practiced being aware of and attuned to God *throughout* your day?

When you're feeling anxious, it's important to have go-to sources of comfort. This can be time with a loved one, quiet time in nature, or reading Scripture. At this moment in your life, what do you find helps calm you?

Hack Your Nervous System

The chemical messengers released from an alarm reaction ignites a call to your body for urgent action, preparing your muscles with the energy necessary to run away from or fight the danger. This explains why it can feel near impossible to attain calm when you're in a state of anxiety. It's like your body is saying, "It's not a time to rest. We're in danger. Get moving!" Your body will not downregulate to calm until it no longer detects danger and returns to safety (with safe people and in a safe environment). However, when you struggle with anxiety, it's like your body is stuck in a cycle of signaling danger. To get unstuck, you need nervous system hacks called vagal tone exercises.

Vagal tone exercises stimulate and strengthen the vagus nerve, which is related to regulating and calming your nervous system. The vagal tone exercises below help you have better mental and physical health. Start by trying one or two of these techniques three to five times a day. Build the habit slowly and stick with it. The investment will pay off in greater concentration, better resilience, and an improved sense of well-being.

- Cold exposure: take a shower, splash your face with cold water, or place a cold compress (like a bag of frozen peas) on your chest.
- Moderate exercise: 30 to 60 minutes of walking, dancing, riding your bike, or jogging.
- Socializing/laughing with people who help you feel safe and comfortable.
- Gargle loudly for 20 to 30 seconds.
- Sing or hum for 2 minutes.

As you complete each task, record your thoughts here about the experience.

Come to me, all you who are weary and burdened, and I will give you rest. Take my yoke upon you and learn from me, for I am gentle and humble in heart, and you will find rest for your souls.

MATTHEW 11:28–29 (NIV)

Praise, worship, fellowship, and time are all exercises that stimulate a rest and restore response. No wonder many people feel so much better after praise, worship, and fellowship time. Think of how this applies to you and describe how spending time with God, in worship and prayer, provides you with peace, comfort, and strength.

Mindful Mornings with God

Have you ever experienced a time when a friend attempted to get your attention by saying, "Hello, I'm right here!" and you replied, "Oh yes! I'm so sorry, I was totally lost in thought!" The same can happen where God is concerned. It is easy to become distracted and not notice that God is with you. Practicing mindful time with God offers opportunity to grow your faith as you move away from mental rumination and into the presence of and communion with God.

Before you get up in the morning, take five minutes to be still with God.

1. Direct your full attention and whole being to the presence of God. Think of His name, His love, His promise of hope, and His blessings and provisions; also think about your gratitude, and love for God, or just be still, aware of God's presence, and listen.

2. When intrusive thoughts interrupt, say, "Stop. I'm busy right now. I'm spending time with God."

3. Then redirect your attention back to being still and focused on God.

4. Redirect your focus as many times as necessary.

5. The goal is to bring your awareness and focus on only one thing in the moment, and that is God.

How did your first mindful morning moment with God feel to you? Write about your experience—what you liked about it, and what you didn't. Then come up with three new ideas for the next time you spend a five-minute moment with God.

The Bible teaches that God holds such great love and compassion for your struggles. If you could talk to God today about your struggles, what would you say, and how would you want Him to respond? Be specific.

"For I know the plans I have for you," declares the Lord, *"plans to prosper you and not to harm you, plans to give you hope and a future."*

JEREMIAH 29:11 (NIV)

Jeremiah 29:11 is a reminder that God does not have plans to harm you but plans to give you a future and provide you with hope. There is so much comfort and strength in this promise! Is there a specific verse that gives you peace and hope? Why?

Radical acceptance is the act of accepting that situations are outside of your control. It does not mean you approve, give permission to, allow, or give up on the situation.

It's been shown to reduce feelings of shame, guilt, and anxiety and break the cycle of bitterness, anger, unhappiness, and suffering. Think of radical acceptance as a way to put your faith into action by releasing what you cannot control over to God and letting God manage what you cannot. What areas in your life have you been assuming control over that you need to release to God?

___

___

___

___

___

___

___

___

___

___

___

___

Practice Radical Acceptance

For this exercise, find a quiet room. Sit in a comfortable position.

1. Think about something you're currently resisting. You'll likely hear yourself say, "I hate, why, if only, should've, would've, could've, I wish . . ."

2. Ask yourself these two questions:

    a. "Is this something I control?"

    b. "Can I change this?"

3. If it is something you can change, and it is wise and best for you to do so, then take proper action.

4. If it is out of your control, then radically accept using this prayer:

   God, I don't like this situation, and I wish it was different, but I acknowledge and accept that I do not have the power to change or control it; it is what it is. I now give it to You to manage and intervene. Give me wisdom, peace, and comfort while navigating through this situation and Your strength to radically accept that which is out of my control. Thank You, Lord.

Many times anxiety is attempting to control the unknown and solve problems it can't solve at the moment. You will recognize this attempt when you find yourself ruminating on a problem or situation it can't resolve in the moment. For example, ruminating over when you will receive the call, what job you will get, what your test results will say. In what situations in your life is your anxiety attempting to control the unknown or solve a problem it can't solve?

The Request Behind the Protest

Behind a protest is a request. For example, when someone says, "You never help me wash the dishes!" the request is, "Will you wash the dishes tonight?" To communicate effectively, turn your protests into requests. The same is true for anxiety. Anxiety is a messenger that is asking you to take appropriate action.

Anxiety frequently protests with "what ifs." The following are a few examples of how you can turn the protest message of "what if" into the matching request for action:

PROTEST	REQUEST
What if I don't have enough money?	I would like to develop a financial plan for…
What if I fail?	I need to develop a plan B if it doesn't work out.
What if I get sick?	I need a plan in the event I get sick.

Learn to better manage your anxiety by decoding the request behind the protest. Now it is your turn. Reframe as many "what if" protests that you can think of into action requests.

PROTEST	REQUEST

In this section, you explored some methods to achieve greater peace. Polyvagal exercises, daily time with God, radical acceptance, and uncovering the requests behind anxieties will all help remove the psychological obstacles that inhibit spiritual growth. These practices will also help you tap into the healing power of your faith. Reflecting on what you've learned, what resonated with you?

_____

_____

_____

_____

_____

_____

_____

_____

_____

_____

_____

_____

_____

_____

_____

_____

_____

11

Challenge Negative Thinking with Biblical Wisdom

P icture this scenario. Person #1 says, "Don't look over there!" Person #2 says, "Where?" and turns to look. It's human nature. Person #1 was focusing on where not to look, and that is where they both ended up looking. The same occurs with thinking. If you focus on the negative, you will perceive and experience more negative, and vice versa with the positive. Scripture provides instruction for where you should place your focus, and psychology has demonstrated that focus is critical to emotional well-being. In this section, you will explore replacing negative thought patterns, which accompany and propel anxiety, with positive thought patterns, using both faith-based and therapeutic practices.

So I say, walk by the Spirit, and you will not gratify the desires of the flesh.

GALATIANS 5:16 (NIV)

Galatians 5:16 states that if you "walk by the Spirit" you won't "gratify the desires of the flesh." When you move toward something, you are not moving toward the opposite—you're not turning left if you're turning right. Now, apply this principle to your mindset. Reframe your mindset from what you don't want (resistance mindset) toward what you do want (forward-focused mindset). Write down a desired outcome you want to achieve, and write it from a forward-focused mindset. For example, "I don't want to be anxious" (resistant mindset), is reframed into a forward-focused mindset: "I want to feel peace. I am learning ways to soothe my nervous system."

Let's continue on with your forward-focused mindset. Know that whatever you focus on is what you move toward. Think for a minute about what you focus on in your life. Once you've got a few ideas in your mind, ask yourself if your thoughts and words and actions are aligned to support what you want in your life. Write your reflections.

Good Thoughts for Well-Being

When your anxious brain is hyper focused on the negative, you can use this verse for guidance on how to redirect your thoughts for emotional well-being. Try your best to acknowledge the truth of what you are experiencing and feeling, with an understanding that remaining in that place can be sticky.

To help your distress tolerance, use this tool to redirect your focus from dwelling on the negative to focusing on God's love and the blessings in your life.

1. Take five minutes and contemplate Philippians 4:8.
2. You can do this sitting in your home or outside on a walk.
3. Reflect on what is true, noble, right, pure, lovely, admirable, excellent, and praiseworthy.
4. Write the verse on an index card and carry it with you. It will remind you to reclaim and live out your life with love, hope, faith, and gratefulness in the full blessings and love that God has for you!

Finally, brothers and sisters, whatever is true, whatever is noble, whatever is right, whatever is pure, whatever is lovely, whatever is admirable—if anything is excellent or praiseworthy—think about such things.

PHILIPPIANS 4:8 (NIV)

You are wonderful, lovely, and admirable. With warts and all, you are incredible, perfectly imperfect. How does Philippians 4:8 help you to challenge negative thinking? What are some warts that you can celebrate rather than worry about?

Negative bias is a tendency not only to notice negative things but also to dwell on the negative. Ruminating on the negative takes a toll on your mental health. Taking steps to elevate your thoughts is a great way to combat negative bias and boost your mood. Take some time to put Philippians 4:8 into action by writing out the answers to these questions:

What are some of your honorable (fine personal) qualities?

What is lovely (pleasing) in your life?

What qualities about you are praiseworthy?

Name some events that have happened in your life that are praiseworthy.

Expand Your Filtering

What you focus on is what you see. This is also called filtering, and it's what can keep you in negative thought patters. This practice will help you mediate your filtering thinking error so you can have a more balanced perspective about your life and achievements.

Set aside fifteen minutes to reflect on your filtering. When you've finished the exercise, write about your experience.

1. Observe what your mind is focusing on. State it out loud with the phrase "I notice . . ." For example, "I notice my thoughts are focusing on what is wrong with this person."

2. Now, turn your mind to notice opposing information.

    a. What is "right" with this person?

    b. What are some of their good qualities?

    c. What are they doing well?

    d. What different things can you notice about them?

    e. What else can you notice or focus on in this moment that is positive?

3. Challenge yourself to get a different perspective.

    a. What can you talk about that is different?

    b. What different things can you do? (Take a different route home?)

4. Diversify your world with new experiences, routines, foods, activities, etc. Introducing new things is healthy for your brain!

Write about your experience here:

Your brain's circuitry, called neural pathways, is established in large part by your thinking habits. The more you think a thought, the stronger the pathway becomes. When a pathway is formed through positive thinking, it can yield benefits in your life. However, when a pathway is grounded in negative thinking, it can distort your perception of yourself and the world around you. But you can undo these pathways. Thankfully, you can create helpful new pathways by repeatedly engaging in positive thinking. To begin rewiring your mind, you must first identify frequent negative thoughts that have become habits. I call these thoughts "stinkin' thinkin'." Take a few minutes to think about your frequent negative thoughts. They can be about yourself, others, your body, opportunities, money, health. Write them here:

Daily Questions to Rewire your Subconscious

Your subconscious holds your internal beliefs about yourself and the world around you. These beliefs are not always accurate or honest or true. What's more, they influence your feelings, responses, and focus. This technique reprograms the belief system in your conscious and subconscious mind. It's not about denying your feelings. Rather, it's about helping you be intentional about what and where you direct your attention. Think of it as rewiring for internal peace.

Ask yourself the following questions every day for the next two weeks. Make note of any feelings or changes that occur within you and your outlook.

- "Why am I so happy?"
- "Why am I so successful?"
- "Why do so many good things happen to me?"
- "Why do I keep attracting good people into my life?"

Do not conform to the pattern of this world, but be transformed by the renewing of your mind. Then you will be able to test and approve what God's will is—his good, pleasing and perfect will.

ROMANS 12:2 (NIV)

When you transform your mind, you turn from your own understanding and begin to take on God's understanding. You adopt God's mindset: to see as God sees, to understand as God understands, and to know what God knows. How would adopting God's mindset change your negative views?

What strengths, qualities, and characteristics do you notice in yourself? Are you having a challenging time generating personal attributes? Ask some supportive and encouraging people that you know what strengths, qualities, etc. they see in you. Write them down to reflect on.

Stop Stinkin' Thinkin' in Its Tracks

This skill is used to check whether your emotional reaction to an event fits the facts of the event or situation. It is especially helpful when emotions are triggered by thought distortions and irrational thinking (stinkin' thinkin') based on assumptions and perceptions of the activating event.

Use your example from the prompts on page 36 to sort through the emotions that are tied to your stinkin' thinkin'.

What is the event/situation prompting my emotion?

Example: You texted your friend, and they did not respond.

What are my thoughts, assumptions, and/or interpretations of the prompting situation?

Assumption: "They're mad at me." "They're ignoring me!"

To detect stinkin' thinkin', ask yourself: Is this statement verified? Is it consistent with known facts?

Unverified: They did not confirm they are mad or intentionally ignoring you.

Verified: They told you they are mad at you and are ignoring you on purpose.

Personal narratives often reinforce negative bias. *Re-storytelling*, from a different perspective, can help replace negative thought patterns with positive thought patterns. Pick one of your personal stories that you typically tell with a negative narrative and rewrite that story from a positive perspective. What went well? What were your highlights, successes, blessings, helpful lessons, etc.?

Let's take a closer look at how your environment affects your mental health. How you live and what you surround yourself with has significant impact on your physical and mental well-being. Take a moment and think about your environment, who you spend time with, what you watch on TV, how much time you spend on social media, etc. Are you ingesting more negativity than positivity? What steps will you take to improve your inputs?

What takeaways from this chapter have helped redirect your negative thoughts? How are you feeling about your abilities in redirecting your negative thoughts? How is your faith involved in these efforts?

III

Nurture your Emotional & Physical Well-Being

To better understand, manage, and break the stigma of anxiety, it's important to recognize that anxiety is biophysiological first and psychological second. This means, experiencing anxiety is part of the body's stress response—an involuntary, unconscious reaction that begins with the input of sensory information. Your conscious brain will then interpret the physiological cues based on prior knowledge, experiences, and expectations. Both your physical reactions and cognitive processes are significantly impacted by diet, physical activity, and environmental variables. In this section, you will explore the mind-body connection while looking at simple steps to manage anxiety through a healthy lifestyle.

So do not fear, for I am with you; do not be dismayed, for I am your God. I will strengthen you and help you; I will uphold you with my righteous right hand.

ISAIAH 41:10 (NIV)

There are three types of anxiety: physical (rapid heart rate, increased blood pressure, headache, rapid breathing, etc.), cognitive (worried thoughts), and spiritual (fearful and worried thoughts of spiritual forces, being abandoned by God). Given the different ways anxiety can be manifested, what kind of fear do you think the Bible is referring to in verses that say "do not fear"? How would you make the distinction between physical fear and cognitive fear?

An overwhelming amount of anxiety, or a constant presence of it, may cause you to struggle with your physical health. How has your anxiety affected your health? What are three changes you'd like to make this week to support your physical health?

How does your physical health affect your mental health and mood? What do you notice is different about you when you're in good health (balanced healthy diet, regular exercise, and sufficient sleep) versus poor health (eating poorly, little to no exercise, poor sleep)?

A cheerful heart is good medicine, but a crushed spirit dries up the bones.

PROVERBS 17:22 (NIV)

Proverbs 17:22 points out how your emotional state can affect your body's health. Do you notice your immune system goes down when you are stressed? What physical symptoms do you experience with an anxious mood? How does your mood affect your health?

Was there a time in your life when you had fun engaging in physical activity? What was the activity? What made it enjoyable? Make some time to journal about how you could begin to incorporate this or other physical activities into your lifestyle.

Nutrition affects your emotional resiliency. What do you notice about the relationship between food and anxiety in your life? Do sugar, caffeine, or other substances make it worse? Do you find you become agitated when you eat salty food? Make some notes about your observations, and pay attention to your emotional responses to nutrition to help manage anxiety.

Keep Calm and Hydrate On

Multiple studies link dehydration with higher risk of anxiety. It is recommended by the Academy of Nutrition and Dietetics to drink between nine and twelve cups of water a day. Amounts vary depending on age, activity level, body mass, and diet.

Boost your water intake this week by setting an alarm to remind you to drink water.

Determine your recommended water intake as follows:

1. Multiply your body weight (in pounds) by 0.5.
2. The result is the number of fluid ounces that you should be drinking per day.
3. Divide the total number of fluid ounces by 8 to arrive at the number of cups.

Your water intake amount is: _____

Use this chart to track your water intake for the week.

	1 CUP	2 CUPS	3 CUPS	4 CUPS	5 CUPS	6 CUPS	7 CUPS	8 CUPS	GOAL MET?
SUN									
MON									
TUE									
WED									
THUR									
FRI									
SAT									

Write about your experience staying hydrated this week.

The Spirit and the bride say, "Come!" And let the one who hears say, "Come!" Let the one who is thirsty come; and let the one who wishes take the free gift of the water of life.

REVELATION 22:17 (NIV)

In Scripture, water symbolizes faith, salvation, and God's provisions. Knowing how essential water is to life, what does Revelation 22:17 mean to you?

Support Your Psychological Immune System

Just as your body has ways of fighting off viruses to improve your physical health, your mind has ways of maintaining your emotional well-being. Nutrition, sleep habits, emotional care, and social interactions all play a part in fortifying your psychological immune system to protect you from the "virus" of negative emotional states.

Set aside time this week to strengthen your psychological immune system. Focus on one of the listed areas each day this week, and mark your progress in the following chart. Repeat next week, but switch up the one you emphasize on each day. After two weeks of emphasis, make an effort to abide by each of them within a given week, as often as possible.

- Practice good sleep hygiene; try to get eight hours of sleep on a regular schedule.
- Focus on eating at regular times with good nutrition. Reduce or avoid sugar, caffeine, and alcohol.
- Exercise once a day.
- Enjoy quality time with loved ones.

	SLEEP	WHOLE FOODS	REDUCE SUGAR, ETC.	EXERCISE
SUN				
MON				
TUE				
WED				
THUR				
FRI				
SAT				

Write any notes here about your week of practicing good sleep hygiene.

_____

_____

_____

_____

_____

_____

Movement Is Medicine

Twenty minutes of daily exercise is as therapeutic as psychotropic medication. Make a commitment to move your body every day for twenty minutes. It doesn't have to be a hard workout that you dread! Focus on activities that you enjoy.

Circle which activities you would enjoy doing:

Walking	Kayaking	Marital Arts
Dancing	Exercise class	Swimming
Rock Climbing	Biking	Paddleboarding
Hiking	Swinging	Roller Skating

Pick two from this list to do this week, and write about your experience in completing them.

_____

_____

_____

_____

_____

_____

_____

_____

It's no secret that many of us live sedentary lives. Think about how much time you spend moving and sitting in one day. Before you go to bed, write down your hours here. Take some more time to reflect on the ratio between your active and inactive lives and what changes you'd like to make for a more active lifestyle.

Tame the Telephone!

Practicing digital hygiene helps reduce anxiety and supports nervous system recovery. When you replace face-to-face communication with face-to-screen communication (texting, social media use, etc.), your brain will automatically activate the fight or flight response. This is a big problem for an overactive, anxious brain! To help the overstimulated nervous system recover, your brain requires human contact with those who help you feel safe.

To help tame anxiety and soothe your nervous system, disconnect from technology, and connect in the human ways your brain understands. To practice digital hygiene this week, give the following a try:

- Before you begin to text someone, make a call instead, or better yet, visit in person.
- Ensure you have daily face-to-face interaction with people you enjoy and trust.
- Put your phone away in the evening and take the week off from social media.

What have you learned about nurturing your emotional and physical health? What takeaways can you incorporate long-term? What practices will you be able to integrate into your daily life to boost your physical and psychological immunity? How do you feel about making these changes?

IV

Look Beyond Prayer for Relief

Years ago, I participated in a Christian diet program that encouraged us to "pray away the pounds." I followed the program as directed, asked for delivery, and prayed my little heart away. Unfortunately, my prayers did not result in one pound of weight loss. Not. One. Pound. I went to the doctor and discovered that my thyroid wasn't creating enough thyroid hormone. That was when I realized God answered my prayers by sending me to the doctor.

Prayer is powerful and necessary, but it is not the only solution. God has provided many resources, both spiritual and physical, that can help manage anxiety. In this section, you will discover new strategies to manage anxiety through faith- and evidence-based practices that align with Christianity.

And in abundance of counselors there is victory.

PROVERBS 24:6 (NASB)

How does the thought of asking for help make you feel? Does it sound like fun or nerve-racking? Does it make you feel weak or strong? How would you do it? Explain your reasonings here.

It isn't always easy to do, but there is no shame in asking for help or requesting some support. Nobody can make it through life alone. Everyone needs help and support in various capacities and at different times. What area in your life do you need more support in right now?

There is a time for everything, and a season for every activity under the heavens.

ECCLESIASTES 3:1 (NIV)

Make Worry Appointments

Worry appointments are designed to help decrease persistent and unwelcome worries. A worry appointment is a time you set aside to exclusively worry. The main benefit comes during the rest of the day, where worry is off limits.

Schedule a worry appointment to exclusively worry. Devote your full attention and energy to nothing but worrying for ten minutes.

DO:

- Stand in front of a mirror and worry out loud.
- Watch and hear yourself worry. (This will help you observe your worry from a different perspective.)
- Worry to the best of your ability.

DON'T:

- Try to change it, minimize your worry, reassure yourself, reason, or relax.
- After ten minutes are up, worrying is off limits. If the worry comes when you're "off worry duty," remind yourself that it will have to wait until your next worry appointment.

Earlier on, you completed an exercise about finding the request behind the protest (page 21). Let's take this a step further by mapping out how a problem can be solved. Pick one of your habitual worries and write out your plan for solving the problem. Use this space to map out your solution. HINT: Your solution may require radical acceptance.

I AM SO WORRIED ABOUT

WHAT I CAN DO ABOUT IT IS

WHAT I CAN'T DO ABOUT IT IS

I CAN BEGIN BY TAKING THESE STEPS

When you're feeling stressed out both emotionally and physically, turning to a trusted friend or family member can help. Who do you turn to for support and why?

Unrealistic expectations and "should" can propel your anxiety. Beliefs such as "I should be able to do this myself," or "I'm weak if I can't handle this," are examples of harmful, unrealistic beliefs. Take time to examine some of your harmful expectations and shoulds, and then write a self-supportive message, making a commitment to releasing them.

SHOULDS	REFRAMING SUPPORTIVE MESSAGE
"I will look stupid if I ask questions."	"I release this belief. It's okay to ask questions. If someone criticizes me, that's their problem, not mine. I give myself full permission to ask."

Now it's your turn.

There is no fear in love. But perfect love drives out fear, because fear has to do with punishment. The one who fears is not made perfect in love.

1 JOHN 4:18 (NIV)

Random Acts of Kindness

Neuroscience has shed light on the teaching "perfect love drives out fear." Loving and kind relationships help down-regulate the nervous system from a fight or flight state to a resting, calm state. Random acts of kindness can lighten your spirit by moving beyond immediate preoccupation with your own concerns and free you from fear. Generosity helps you overcome separation and can reconnect you with someone.

Take a look at the list here, and then add your own random acts of kindness you can do this week. Make sure to complete one at least every day.

- Be present for someone
- Buy someone a coffee
- Smile at someone
- Give a hug
- Make something for someone
- Put money in someone's parking meter
- Volunteer
- _____
- _____
- _____
- _____
- _____

- _____
- _____
- _____
- _____
- _____
- _____
- _____
- _____
- _____

So, how did it feel to practice random acts of kindness? How did people respond? How did their feelings affect your feelings? What are your feelings when you do random acts of kindness without recognition? Write down the things you observed from extending your generosity.

Think of someone who made you feel grounded and calm when you were distressed. What attributes or actions of theirs helped you feel grounded? How could you draw inspiration from the example they set the next time you are distressed? Write out how you will commit to doing that.

Four Square Breathing

Deep breathing stimulates the parasympathetic nervous system—your calm state. If you're new to breathing exercises, you might get a little dizzy. If this happens, stop, remain seated, and wait until you're not dizzy, and then begin again.

Start in the upper left corner, and trace your finger along the lines as you breathe.

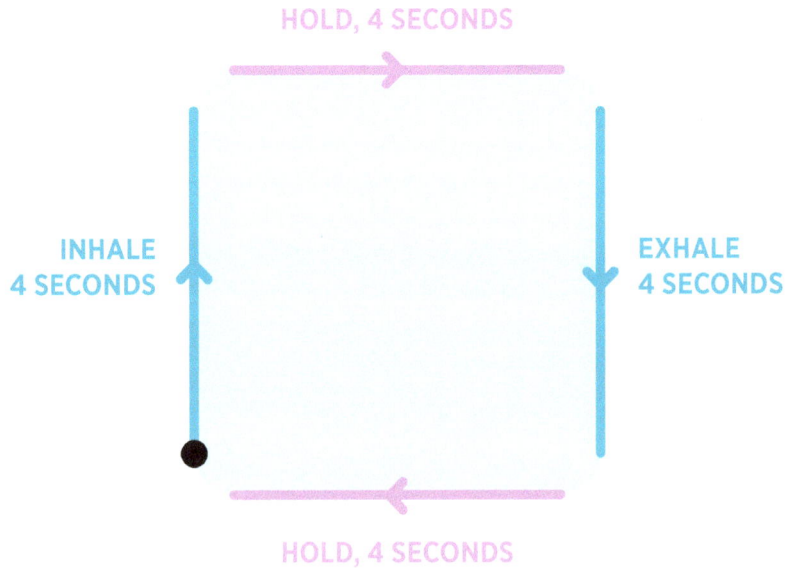

Set your alarm to remind yourself when to practice. When you breathe, concentrate on breathing with your diaphragm. Before you begin, find a safe, quiet, stress-free environment to practice in and focus on your breathing.

1. Sit down and place your hands on your lap, palms up.
2. Slowly exhale, getting all the oxygen out of your lungs.
3. Slowly inhale for a count of four (count very slowly in your head). Let the air move into your abdomen.
4. Hold your breath for a slow count of four.
5. Exhale through your mouth for a slow count of four.
6. Repeat the process four times.

5-4-3-2-1 Grounding for Anxiety

Grounding exercises use mental distractions to help reduce distressing feelings and redirect your focus from the distress, back to the here and now.

Use this grounding technique for anxiety. Focus on:

- 5 things you see around you (name them out loud or in your mind)
- 4 things you can touch/feel (something soft, hard, smooth—what can you find?)
- 3 things you can hear (in the room, outside, in your body)
- 2 things you can smell
- 1 thing you can taste

Now that you've experienced and practiced a number of different grounding techniques, how did that resonate with you? What did you like? What didn't you enjoy? How do you plan to incorporate more grounding techniques in your day?

V

Self-Care through God's Love

Think about how it feels when a loved one takes good care of themselves or when they don't. Of course, you want those you love to value their lives and care for their health. God desires the same for you. In fact, Scripture teaches that your body is a valuable temple of the Holy Spirit. You can't get more valuable than that!

Yet many women have been taught that if they spend time on looking or feeling good they are being vain, selfish, prideful, etc. It's time to break this problematic perspective! Taking care of yourself not only glorifies God and honors the gift He gave you, but it is also essential for managing anxiety. This section will give you an opportunity to explore self-care and self-love strategies to support anxiety management.

Love is patient, love is kind. It does not envy, it does not boast, it is not proud. It does not dishonor others, it is not self-seeking, it is not easily angered, it keeps no record of wrongs. Love does not delight in evil but rejoices with truth.

1 CORINTHIANS 13:4–6 (NIV)

Many people struggle with the concept of self-love. They presume they must first feel self-love to begin to love themselves. Based on 1 Corinthians 13, do you believe that love is a feeling, an action, or both? Can you love yourself without feeling love?

What about the term *self-care*? What were you taught about self-care? How does it relate to self-love, and how is it related to your relationship with God?

Using 1 Corinthians 13:4–6 as inspiration, write a declaration of self-love to yourself. Start from the prompt here.

"I will be patient and kind to myself. I will not allow myself to compare myself to others or seek outside approval."

Even though Corinthians provides guidance to not keep a record of wrongs, the anxious brain often does the opposite by maintaining and ruminating on a running list of everything you feel you've done wrong. What worries and intrusive thoughts keep you up at night or are constantly in the forefront of your mind? Take inventory by writing down some of the items on your mind's running list.

Practice Kindsight

Kindsight is a self-compassionate way to frame and think about failures, mistakes, and regrets. It looks for the helpful lessons and insights gained from your past experiences and does not get stuck in self-critical rumination. Kindsight will help you manage your anxiety as it is not threatened by making mistakes and offers self-support and compassion.

Practice reframing hindsight into kindsight.

Hindsight: "What was I thinking? I should have chosen the other one!"

Reframed Kindsight: "I did not think of that at the time. If it ever happens again, I will choose the other one."

Now, look back at your list from the previous prompt on page 92 and pick a few of your regrets or critical ruminations regarding previous choices, behaviors, or mistakes, and convert them into kindsight statements. Reframe them with a kind, supportive voice. Use phrases like, "I learned from . . . I am now aware . . . in the future I will . . ." Write them down here:

_____

_____

_____

_____

_____

_____

_____

_____

Above all else, guard your heart, for everything you do flows from it.

PROVERBS 4:23 (NIV)

Part of caring for and loving yourself is noticing and celebrating what you have done well. Take time now to reflect on and write down something you recently did well. What can you do this week to celebrate success?

Pretend your best friend has just come to you with an issue that was created by her own doing. She's doing a great job of beating herself up. What would you tell her to make her feel a little bit better? Now apply this principle to yourself and be your own best friend. Encourage yourself and write down your best attributes here.

Practice Self-Compassion

Now it's time to take that same compassion that you showed your friend and apply it to yourself. Practice goodwill toward yourself, radically accepting your struggles and at the same time embracing yourself with kindness and care, remembering you are part of the shared human experience. In many ways it's the ultimate form of self-care.

Set aside thirty minutes to practice self-compassion. If you aren't used to self-compassion, it may feel awkward at first, but as you practice you'll find it easier to do.

Some ideas for self-compassion include:

Treat yourself as you would treat a good friend. Give yourself the tenderness and care you need when you're going through a tough time.

Example: On a stressful day, make some warm tea or soup, wrap up in a comfy blanket, snuggle up on your couch, and turn on your favorite show or read your favorite book.

Communicate understanding and patience to yourself regarding your own struggles and perceived flaws with positive self-talk.

Example: "Even though I am struggling with anxiety, I completely love and accept myself."

Accept your imperfect human condition with empathy and thoughtfulness, and give yourself a pep talk.

Example: "Being human is tough. Struggling is a normal part of life, and I am not alone; God understands and loves me just the way I am, and does not expect me to be perfect."

Describe how God may feel when you take care of yourself. How would it delight and please Him to see you valuing yourself and honoring your identity as His child? Why would that be important to God?

Anticipate Your Needs

Self-care involves proactively anticipating and planning for your present and future needs like a parent who prepares for their child's needs (carrying snacks, making sure the child has a nap, planning play dates, going to the doctor, etc.). Planning and being prepared and present help a child feel safe and secure.

Be your best inner parent by proactively attending to your daily and future needs. Pick something from the following list (or generate your own ideas). Pick a new one each week.

- Plan your nutritional needs and food for the day. Have snacks on hand and pack your meals for when you are at work or on the go.
- Begin a savings account for your dream vacation.
- Schedule time to rest. Take a nap or just lie down during the day so you can restore your physical and mental health.
- _____
- _____
- _____
- _____
- _____
- _____
- _____
- _____
- _____

Create Positive Emotions with Enjoyable Activities

One holiday I found myself completely burned out and lost all joy for cooking . . . until I decided to cook something special just for myself. Suddenly, cooking became fun again! Making something special for myself lifted my spirits and brought energy back into my body and joy into my day. You too can boost your mood by finding ways to create positive emotions with enjoyable activities.

Chose two enjoyable activities, one for each week, that you will commit to over the next two weeks. You can choose from those provided or come up with your own ideas.

- Take a bubble bath
- Massage your scalp as you shampoo
- Put on lotion after a bath
- Give yourself a pedicure and manicure
- Play outdoors (e.g., kayaking, paddleboarding!)
- Read uplifting literature
- _____
- _____
- _____
- _____

- _____
- _____
- _____
- _____
- _____
- _____
- _____
- _____

What activities generate positive feelings for you? They can be as simple as repotting your favorite plant, baking your favorite treat, or even completing a nagging task like cleaning out your garage. Make a list, and then commit to completing one of them each month.

For you created my inmost being; You knit me together in my mother's womb. I praise you because I am fearfully and wonderfully made.

PSALM 139:13–14 (NIV)

To help transform your mental habit of focusing on what's "wrong with me?" you must train your brain to focus on *what's right with you*. To recognize the qualities and gifts that you possess. What are some of the personal qualities you appreciate about your unique design? Knowing that you are God's treasure, what three things will you do this week to take special care of God's gift that is YOU?

VI

Calm Anxiety with a Grateful Heart

Gratitude is more than a mindset, mental discipline, or a display of virtue. It is a superpower to defeat your enemies and fill you with hope and joy. Embracing and practicing gratitude on a regular basis can lift your mood, improve mental health, reduce stress, improve nervous system health, and strengthen emotional resiliency, all while fulfilling a core tenet of your faith. This section will focus on the practice of gratitude and how you can use this superpower to aid in the struggle with anxiety.

Do not be anxious about anything, but in everything by prayer and pleading with thanksgiving let your requests be made known to God. And the peace of God, which surpasses all comprehension, will guard your hearts and your minds in Christ Jesus.

PHILIPPIANS 4:6-7 (NASB)

What is the connection between thanksgiving, peace, and your heart and mind, as talked about in Philippians 4:6-7? Why is it so important?

How often do you express gratitude throughout your day? Is the gratitude expressed to someone? To God? What makes expressing gratitude easy for you? What makes it hard?

Daily Delight Practice

Your brain is hardwired to selectively focus on what's wrong. This is referred to as negative bias. *To combat this tendency, you can train your brain to develop an optimistic outlook by intentionally focusing attention on your positive experiences.*

For this practice, your objective is to notice and hold gratitude for simple everyday experiences. This can include a smile, a kind act, time with your pets, or something in nature. To begin the practice of being aware of gratitude throughout your day, pause and notice what you might be grateful for during your transitions throughout the day:

Notice something you are grateful for:

- When you wake up
- When you leave your house in the morning
- During mealtimes
- When you go on an errand
- When you return home
- As you prepare to go to sleep
- _____
- _____
- _____
- _____
- _____
- _____
- _____
- _____
- _____
- _____
- _____
- _____

You can increase the effects of gratitude by sharing gratitude with others! Write a gratitude letter to someone you appreciate or who has made a difference in your life. After you do, choose whether to share the letter with them. Notice how your mood improves when you share your gratitude with others, even if only on paper, and unbeknownst to them.

Negativity Fast

Your thoughts and words have power, so you can leverage them to maximize your breakthrough. With a negativity fast, you are detoxifying your thinking, speaking, negative mental habits, and relational patterns so that they align with and support the positive outcomes you want to create. Negativity fasts help you develop hopeful patterns, build positive mental habits, improve your mood, and break negative thought loops.

For the next week, practice your negativity fast with these steps:

ABSTAIN FROM:

1. News and social media.
2. Critically talking about yourself and others.
3. Talking about situations and people with a negative viewpoint.
4. Complaining and gossiping.
5. Sarcasm related to negative and bitter views.

INTENTIONALLY FOCUS ON:

1. God's love and goodness.
2. Speaking out thanksgiving and praise.
3. Declaring who God is and who God says you are.
4. Speaking life, love, and hope to ourselves and others.
5. What God is doing, and bring it up in conversation.

ADDITIONAL GUIDELINES:

1. It's okay to cry and have tender emotional moments. The goal is not to add any unnecessary negativity like speaking hopelessness and discouraging talk.

2. Each time you are tempted to criticize someone, immediately pray a blessing for them.

3. Do not criticize others for being negative; avoid judging!

Record your experience here:

...all your ways submit to him, and he will make your paths straight.

PROVERBS 3:5-6 (NIV)

Accepting happiness can make you stronger and more grateful for what you have. It also helps build emotional resiliency and strength for facing difficult times in the future. How easy or difficult is it for you to embrace, acknowledge, and savor happiness? What gets in the way?

Embrace Happiness

Now that you've identified the challenges you feel in embracing your happiness, set aside some time to identify and hold gratitude for the things that are good in you.

Write down three things you are grateful for about yourself in each of the following categories.

PHYSICAL

1. _____
2. _____
3. _____

MENTAL

1. _____
2. _____
3. _____

SPIRITUAL

1. _____
2. _____
3. _____

Counting your blessings really does make a difference. What are five things you are blessed with? Examples include: your ability to spell anything by just hearing the word, having the patience to train your cat to take a bath, or your ability to sniff out insincerity in another person in a matter of seconds. Start each one off with:

"I'm good at . . ."

1. _____

2. _____

3. _____

4. _____

5. _____

Establish the habit of noticing the positive and bringing positive experiences into your conscious awareness. At the end of each day, take a minute to list five things you were grateful to witness, and then write a prayer of gratitude about it.

1.

2.

3.

4.

5.

Practicing gratitude takes practice. Take a few minutes each morning to give thanks for your experiences the day before. Say your gratitude prayer every morning. Develop a prayer of gratitude and write it out here.

Create Your Gratitude Buddies

Gratitude improves your emotional resiliency and shapes your neuropathways to support positive thoughts and emotions. Spending time with a gratitude buddy stimulates the calming effects of your nervous system and strengthens your ventral vagus nerve function, which will help improve your ability to regulate your nervous system.

Find a gratitude partner who will be committed to regularly meeting and expressing gratitude. Set aside time to meet up (phone, coffee, or video chat) and discuss your gratitude. Ask each other questions and share thoughts of gratefulness. This will help you sustain motivation and strengthen your emotional resiliency. Here are some ideas for questions:

- What was the best part of your day?
- What made you smile today?
- Who helped you today?
- Who was kind to you today?
- How are you fortunate?

Distracted by your struggles, you may not notice the support you actually have and the people in your life who are kind and loving. Practicing gratitude for people can help you not take for granted the supportive people in your life. Write about three people you're thankful for today and why. Try to notice the support you receive throughout the day.

Peace I leave you, My peace I give you; not as the world gives, do I give to you. Do not let your heart be troubled, nor fearful.

JOHN 14:27 (NASB)

Think about how your relationship with God has given you peace and hope. Write a thank you note to God describing how your relationship has made a difference in your life.

Continue your Healing Journey with Faith

Congratulations on completing this journal! One of my mentors once said, "Shawn, remember, it's all about the process, not the end result." It is important to remember that healing is not a destination; it is a process. It is more than healing—it is growing, evolving, and transforming. It is the journey of a lifetime. The most amazing part is how God is revealed along the journey and offers you many opportunities to grow closer to Him and deepen your faith.

I hope you found this journal helpful. You can come back to it and continue to use and experience the benefits of these tools over and over again!

Thank you for taking a deep dive with me. I wish you the very best on your journey.

Blessings, my friend!

Shawn Horn, PsyD

NOTES

NOTES

Resources

Podcasts

Inspired Living with Dr. Shawn Horn—Providing encouragement, education, and inspiration for healing, hope, and wholehearted living.

Stronger in the Difficult Places with Dr. Zoe Shaw—Helping women stay strong and transform difficult relationships.

The Faith & Wellness Podcast with Brittney Moses—Integrating faith and mental health for your health and wellness.

Blog

drshawnhorn.com—Inspired Living School, an online self-help education for personal development and growth.

Apps

ABIDE—Pray and Relax biblical meditations to help with sleep and stress reduction.

iChill—An app to help guide you in the use of the Community Resiliency Model, a set of wellness skills. Learn simple information about how stress affects the mind and body.

F&MW—Brittney Moses's faith and mental wellness app for Christian women.

References

Anxiety & Depression Association of America. "Did You Know?" adaa.org/understanding-anxiety/facts-statistics.

Barlow, D. H., and M. G. Craske. *Mastery of Your Anxiety and Panic Workbook* (4th edition). New York: Oxford University Press, 2007.

Berger, Allen. *12 Essential Insights for Emotional Sobriety: Getting Your Recovery Unstuck*. Redondo Beach, CA: 4th Dimension Publishing, 2022.

Chen, Ying, and Tyler J. VanderWeele. "Associations of Religious Upbringing with Subsequent Health and Well-Being from Adolescence to Young Adulthood: An Outcome-Wide Analysis." *American Journal of Epidemiology* 187, no. 11 (2018): 2355–64. doi.org/10.1093/aje/kwy142.

Dana, Deb. *Polyvagal Exercises for Safety and Connection*. New York: W. W. Norton & Company, Inc., 2020.

Linehan, Marsha M. *DBT Skills Training Manual 2nd Edition*. New York: The Guilford Press, 2015.

McKay, M., J. C. Wood, and J. Brantley. *The Dialectical Behavior Therapy Skills Workbook: Practical DBT Exercises for Learning Mindfulness, Interpersonal Effectiveness, Emotion Regulation & Distress Tolerance*. Oakland, CA: New Harbinger Publications, 2007.

Spradlin, S. E. *Don't Let Your Emotions Run Your Life: How Dialectical Behavior Therapy Can Put You in Control*. Oakland, CA: New Harbinger Press, 2003.

Whitley, Rob. "'Thank You God': Religion and Recovery from Dual Diagnosis among Low-Income African Americans." *Transcultural Psychiatry* 49, no. 1 (2011): 87–104. citeseerx.ist.psu.edu /viewdoc/download?doi=10.1.1.972.748&rep=rep1&type=pdf.

Yamada, A.-M., D. Lukoff, C. S. F. Lim, and L. L. Mancuso. "Integrating Spirituality and Mental Health: Perspectives of Adults Receiving Public Mental Health Services in California." *Psychology of Religion and Spirituality*, 12, no.3 (2020): 276–87. doi.org/10.1037 /rel0000260.

Acknowledgments

Thank you to my colleagues for their fantastic support: Rita Flanagan, Rich Wilson, Beth Fitterer, Therese Mascardo, Diane Strachowski, Sophie Mort, Hayden Finch, Zoe Shaw, Marie Fang, and my "psychology squad." To my mentors who guided me through different stages of my career: Kathryn Ecklund, Nancy Thurston, Carol Del'Oliver and Kathleen Gathercoal. To Marsha Linehan, Stephen Porges, and Deb Dana for their research and work.

Finally, to my family and friends for their endless love and support: Joel, Jacob and Sarah Horn, Diann and TJ Knowles, Paul and Sally Ayer, Eldon and Meri Horn, Deann Ayer, Debbie Dautel, Janet Henson, Vanessa Gibson, Marti and Eddie Horn, and Brooklynn Graham.

About the Author

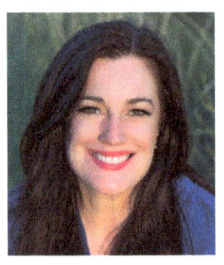

Shawn Horn, PsyD, is a licensed clinical psychologist, author, podcast host, and TEDx speaker. In addition to her private practice, she serves as clinical supervisor for the University of Washington–affiliated psychiatric residency program, is host of *Inspired Living Podcast*, and is an expert contributor to *Uncovered: Stories of Shame & Struggle with Nichole Mischke*. With over two decades of experience in the mental health field, she is now bringing the wisdom of the therapy room to you with her online Inspired Living School, where she helps students heal from shame and acquire skills for emotional resiliency and wholehearted living. Follow her on social media @drshawnhorn.